Multiple True/False Questions for the Primary FRCA:
Physiology and Anatomy

Simon A. May

CONTENTS

INTRODUCTION

At the time of writing, the MCQ component of the Primary FRCA examination comprises 90 multiple choice questions, to be completed within 3 hours. 30 of these questions are single best answer (SBA) questions and the remaining 60 questions are multiple true/false (MTF) questions. The MTF questions are designed to test theoretical knowledge, whereas the SBA questions will require you to apply this knowledge.

The 60 MTF questions are subdivided, approximately, as follows:
- 20 MTF questions in pharmacology
- 20 MTF questions in physiology and anatomy
- 20 MTF questions in physics, clinical measurement and data interpretation.

Each MTF question consists of a stem followed by 5 statements, each of which requires a true or false answer.

The questions in this book are based on the knowledge required for the MTF physiology and anatomy component of the Primary FRCA MCQ exam. The SBA and other MTF components of the Primary FRCA MCQ exam are covered in separate books in the *Revise Anaesthesia* series.

The breadth and style of the questions mirror the Primary FRCA MCQ exam and for each question, there is a concise explanation. The questions are arranged into groups of 20 questions, followed by the answers and explanations for those questions.

MCQ books are an essential aid to FRCA exam revision. They quickly identify gaps in knowledge and therefore help focus future revision. The *Revise Anaesthesia* series differs from other MCQ books, as you are able to purchase questions separately for each component of the exam. This allows the books to be used as part of topic-specific revision and provides an alternative to expensive subscription-based question banks. Available in paperback and e-book format, the questions are yours to keep and access anywhere.

Best of luck in the examinations.

Questions 1-20

Q1:
Regarding the central venous pressure waveform:
A. The "a" wave corresponds to atrial relaxation
B. The "c" wave corresponds to isovolumetric contraction of the ventricle
C. The "v" wave corresponds to closure of the tricuspid valve
D. The "x" descent corresponds to opening of the pulmonary valve
E. The "y" descent corresponds to rapid ventricular filling after opening of the tricuspid valve

Q2:
Regarding the anatomy of the diaphragm:
A. The inferior vena cava traverses the diaphragm at T10
B. The aorta, thoracic duct and azygous vein traverse the diaphragm at the same level
C. Both phrenic nerves pierce the diaphragm
D. The left crura is attached to the first and second lumbar vertebral bodies
E. There are two arcuate ligaments

Q3:
Regarding anatomical and physiological dead space:
A. Anatomical dead space increases with deep inspiration
B. Fowler's method can be utilised to measure physiological dead space
C. Fowler's method requires the measurement of expiratory carbon dioxide
D. The Bohr equation assumes all carbon dioxide is derived from alveolar gas
E. In lung disease, physiological and anatomical dead space volumes are equal

Q4:

Regarding the metabolic effects of insulin:

A. Increases the rate of protein synthesis
B. Increases the rate of glycogenolysis
C. Increases the rate of breakdown of triglycerides
D. Increases the rate of ketone body synthesis
E. Increases fatty acid synthesis

Q5:

Regarding the control of bicarbonate by the kidneys:

A. Bicarbonate is freely filtered by the glomerulus
B. 90% of bicarbonate is reabsorbed by the distal nephron
C. Proximal tubular reabsorption of bicarbonate requires carbonic anhydrase
D. Distal tubular reabsorption requires the active transport of hydrogen ions into the tubular fluid
E. Phosphate in the renal tubule inhibits bicarbonate absorption

Q6:

Regarding the Valsalva manoeuvre:

A. It is the forceful expiration of air against an open glottis
B. During phase 1, heart rate reduces
C. During phase 2, heart rate increases
D. An absent overshoot in phase 3 is characteristic of autonomic dysfunction
E. A square wave response is associated with congestive cardiac failure

Q7:
Nicotinic acetylcholine receptors:
A. Have a molecular weight of approximately 250 daltons
B. Consists of 7 polypeptide subunits
C. Protein subunit expression is different between the foetus and adult
D. When open, the channel allows the passage of anions
E. Acetylcholine molecules bind to the beta subunit of the receptor

Q8:
Regarding nerve fibres:
A. A_α fibres have a conduction velocity of 70-120ms^{-1}
B. C fibres are unmyelinated
C. The diameter of a B fibre axon is 18μm
D. Touch and pressure are functions of A_β fibres
E. Preganglionic fibres of the sympathetic nervous system are unmyelinated

Q9:
The following cause a right shift of the oxygen dissociation curve:
A. Increased temperature
B. Increased partial pressure of carbon dioxide
C. Increased levels of 2,3 diphosphoglycerate
D. Acidotic environment
E. Foetal haemoglobin

Q10:
Regarding cardiac pacemaker cell depolarisation:
A. Phase 0 occurs due to calcium ion efflux through T type channels
B. The resting membrane potential is approximately -90mV
C. The threshold potential is approximately -40mV
D. Phase 4 corresponds to the movement of sodium ions out of the cell
E. Phase 2 of the action potential is prolonged compared to cardiac myocytes

Q11:
The following are contained in the male inguinal canal:
A. Genital branch of the genitofemoral nerve
B. Ilioinguinal nerve
C. Pampiniform plexus
D. Round ligament
E. Fascia transversalis

Q12:
Regarding pulmonary vascular resistance:
A. As pulmonary arterial pressure increases, pulmonary vascular resistance falls
B. As pulmonary venous pressure increases, pulmonary vascular resistance falls
C. Pulmonary vascular resistance increases with high lung volumes
D. Pulmonary vascular resistance increases with low lung volumes
E. Acetylcholine increases pulmonary vascular resistance

Q13:

Regarding the composition of gastric fluid:

A. It has the same sodium concentration as plasma
B. It has a higher chloride content than saliva
C. It has the same bicarbonate concentration as bile
D. It has a lower pH than sweat
E. It does not contain potassium

Q14:

Regarding the glomerulus:

A. The glomerular basement membrane has a positive charge
B. The glomerular filtration rate is approximately 180 litres of blood per day
C. Hydrostatic pressure in the glomerular capillary network is higher than the capillary hydrostatic pressure in other organs
D. Colloid osmotic pressure is the same at the afferent and efferent ends of the glomerular capillary network
E. The glomerular capillary is 10 times more permeable than capillaries in other organs

Q15:

Regarding the citric acid (Kreb) cycle:

A. Acetyl-CoA enters the cycle by binding to citrate which forms oxaloacetate
B. Carbon dioxide is produced as a by product of the cycle
C. 1 molecule of acetyl-CoA entering the cycle will produce 3 molecules of NADH
D. A single cycle produces 38 ATP molecules
E. Occurs in the cytosol

Q16:

The following factors increase the rate of gastric emptying:
A. Cholecystokinin
B. Gastrin
C. Motilin
D. Secretin
E. Somatostatin

Q17:

Regarding the foetal circulation:
A. Consists of a single umbilical vein
B. Oxygen saturation in the umbilical artery is approximately 80%
C. Pulmonary vascular resistance is relatively high in the foetus
D. The majority of blood entering the right atrium traverses the foramen ovale
E. Oxygen saturation in the superior vena cava is approximately 75%

Q18:

Regarding thyroid hormone synthesis:
A. Iodide is taken up by thyroid cells via an ATP dependant sodium-iodide pump
B. Thyroid peroxidase catalyses the formation of tri-iodothyronine and tetra-iodothyronine in the thyroid cells
C. Thyroid peroxidase oxidises iodide to iodine
D. The combination of mono-iodothyronine and di-iodothyronine forms tri-iodothyronine
E. Reverse tri-iodothyronine is an inactive substance

Q19:

Regarding pancreatic secretion:

A. 1500ml of pancreatic fluid is produced daily
B. Secretin stimulates the production of large volumes of chloride rich pancreatic fluid
C. Pancreatic secretions have a pH of 2
D. The acini cells secrete trypsin into the pancreatic fluid
E. Bicarbonate is secreted entirely by epithelial cells of the pancreatic ducts

Q20:

Myocardial contractility is increased by:

A. Acidosis
B. Hypoxia
C. Increasing calcium ion concentration
D. Parasympathetic stimulation
E. Sympathetic stimulation

Q1:
A. **F**
B. **T**
C. **F**
D. **T**
E. **T**

The central venous waveform comprises a, c and v waves and an x and y descent.

The "a" waves correspond to atrial contraction.

The "c" waves correspond to isovolumetric contraction of the ventricle.

The "v" waves correspond to the opening of the tricuspid valve.

The "x" descent corresponds to the fall in right ventricular pressure when the pulmonary valve opens.

The "y" descent corresponds to the rapid filling of the ventricle when the tricuspid valve opens.

Q2:

A. F
B. T
C. T
D. T
E. F

The diaphragm consists of three arcuate ligaments (median, medial and lateral) and two crura. The left crura is attached to the first and second vertebral body and the right crura is attached to the first, second and third vertebral bodies.

The inferior vena cava traverses the diaphragm at T8, as does the right phrenic nerve. At T10, the oesophagus, vagus nerve, left gastric artery and vein travel through the diaphragm. At T12, the aorta, thoracic duct and azygous vein traverse the diaphragm.

The left phrenic nerve traverses the diaphragm separately through the muscle.

Q3:

A. T
B. F
C. F
D. T
E. F

Anatomical dead space in the adult is approximately 150ml and is defined as the volume of the conducting airways (i.e. the airways that do not take part in gas exchange). Anatomical dead space increases with deep inspiration due to the traction generated on the airways. Fowler's method allows for the measurement of physiological dead space by recording the subject's end tidal nitrogen concentration against time and assessing when the plateau phase occurs. The Bohr equation is used to derive the physiological dead space, which is the volume of the airways and lung parenchyma that do not take part in gas exchange. In health, physiological and anatomical dead space values are very similar but in diseased states the physiological dead space can exceed anatomical dead space.

Q4:
A. T
B. F
C. F
D. F
E. T

Insulin has the following metabolic effects:
- Increases glycolysis
- Increases glycogen synthesis
- Increases protein synthesis
- Increases fatty acid synthesis
- Decreases glycogenolysis
- Decreases ketone body formation
- Reduces the breakdown of triglyceride

Q5:
A. T
B. F
C. T
D. T
E. F

Bicarbonate is essential in the control of the acid-base balance of the body. Bicarbonate is freely filtered at the glomerulus and is then nearly entirely reabsorbed by the kidney. 90% of bicarbonate reabsorption occurs in the proximal tubule and the remaining 10% occurs in the distal tubule.

Bicarbonate combines with hydrogen ions (which are excreted by the proximal tubule) in the tubular fluid, under the influence of carbonic anhydrase, to form water and carbon dioxide. The carbon dioxide is able to cross the tubular cell membrane and then intracellularly, under the influence of carbonic anhydrase, reforms bicarbonate and hydrogen ions. In the cell, hydrogen ions are then re-circulated into the tubule and bicarbonate is exported back into the plasma. This mechanism occurs in the proximal and distal tubule, but distal tubular hydrogen ion secretion requires more energy due to the reduction in hydrogen ion gradient as the urine acidifies during its journey through the nephron.

As bicarbonate is reabsorbed by the kidney, phosphate can be utilised by the body to act as a buffer for hydrogen ions to enable the continued reabsorption of bicarbonate.

Q6:
A. F
B. T
C. T
D. F
E. T

The Valsalva manoeuvre is the forceful expiration of air against a closed glottis, whereas Müller's manoeuvre is the forceful inspiration of air against a closed nose and mouth after exhalation. The Valsalva manoeuvre plots heart rate and blood pressure against time during which a subject forcefully exhales against a closed glottis.

During phase 1, blood pressure momentarily increases and heart rate decreases.

During phase 2, sympathetic stimulation causes an increase in heart rate and blood pressure.

During phase 3, exhalation is stopped against a closed glottis and blood pressure momentarily falls (with a preserved heart rate).

Finally, in phase 4 an overshoot of blood pressure occurs due to maintained vasoconstriction and a sudden increase in cardiac output. This also causes the heart rate to fall.

An absent overshoot in phase 4 of the valsalva manoeuvre is associated with autonomic dysfunction and a square wave response is associated with congestive cardiac failure.

Q7:
A. F
B. F
C. T
D. F
E. F

The nicotinic acetylcholine receptor (nAChR) has a mass of 250kDa and is expressed on the pre and post synaptic membrane of the neuromuscular junction. It comprises 5 protein subunits. The structure varies between the adult and foetus. The adult receptor has two α, one β, one δ and one ε protein subunits unlike the foetus which has one γ subunit instead of one ε protein subunit. When in the open conformational state, the central pore of the molecule allows the passage of cations not anions. The main cation that traverses this central pore is sodium. Acetylcholine binds to the α-subunit of the receptor.

Q8:

A. T
B. T
C. F
D. T
E. F

- All nerve fibres except C fibres are myelinated.
- A_α fibres have the largest diameter (9-18μm) and have the fastest conduction (at 70-120ms⁻¹). They function as motor fibres and spindle afferents.
- B fibres have a preganglionic function, are myelinated and have a diameter of 3μm.
- C fibres are responsible for the transmission of pain, touch and heat sensation. They have a slow conduction velocity and small axon diameter.
- A_β (touch and pressure), A_γ (motor to muscle spindles) and A_δ (pain, pressure and temperature) are myelinated nerve fibres with intermediate nerve conduction velocities.

Q9:

A. T
B. T
C. T
D. T
E. F

A right shift in the oxygen dissociation curve enhances the ability of the haemoglobin molecule to offload oxygen. This occurs in environments that are acidotic, have an increased temperature, have an increased partial pressure of carbon dioxide or if the body has increased levels of 2,3 diphosphoglycerate (2,3 dpg). Foetal haemoglobin has a different structure to adult haemoglobin. This makes it harder to offload oxygen, therefore, the oxygen dissociation curve for foetal haemoglobin is shifted to the left.

Q10:
A. F
B. F
C. T
D. F
E. F

Cardiac pacemaker cell depolarisation consists of phases 0, 3 and 4 (there is no phase 1 or 2). During phase 0, calcium ions influx through T type channels once the threshold potential has been reached (around -40mV). A depolarisation period then occurs (phase 3) that restores the resting membrane potential, which is around -60mV. During phase 4, spontaneous sodium leakage into the cell causes the resting membrane potential to increase to the threshold potential enabling another action potential to form.

Q11:
A. T
B. T
C. T
D. F
E. F

The male inguinal canal contains the spermatic cord and ilioinguinal nerve. The spermatic cord consists of the vas deferens, testicular artery, cremasteric artery, artery to vas, pampiniform plexus, sympathetic plexus and the genital branch of the genitofemoral nerve.

The female inguinal canal contains the ilioinguinal nerve and round ligament.

The fascia transversalis forms the posterior boundary of the inguinal canal.

Q12:
A. T
B. T
C. T
D. T
E. F

Pulmonary vascular resistance decreases with either increasing venous or increasing arterial pressure. This is because increasing pressure in the pulmonary bed leads to the opening of closed capillaries (recruitment) and the enlargement of already open capillaries (distention). Pulmonary vascular resistance is increased at both low and high lung volumes. At low lung volumes, the increase in pulmonary vascular resistance occurs due to extra-alveolar vessels narrowing. At high volumes, the increased resistance is caused by capillary stretching.

Acetylcholine causes smooth muscle relaxation, therefore reducing pulmonary vascular resistance.

Q13:
A. F
B. T
C. F
D. T
E. F

Gastric fluid has a pH of 3 and contains 60mmoll^{-1} of sodium, 9mmoll^{-1} of potassium, 84mmoll^{-1} of chloride and no bicarbonate. It is more acidic than saliva, bile and sweat.

Gastric fluid has less sodium than plasma, more chloride than saliva (but less than bile) and like saliva and sweat contains no bicarbonate (unlike bile).

Q14:
A. F
B. F
C. T
D. F
E. F

The glomerulus is a capillary network in the kidney which has a filtration rate of approximately 180 litres of plasma per day. It has a glomerular basement membrane which is negatively charged, thus helping to prevent the passage of proteins (e.g. albumin) into the ultrafiltrate. It has pores which enable the free passage of molecules up to 7000 daltons in size (though molecules as large as 70000 daltons can traverse the membrane). As plasma passes through the glomerulus; the muscle tone in the afferent and efferent arterioles maintain the hydrostatic pressure and due to a concentration effect, the colloid osmotic pressure increases as you approach the efferent arteriole. Compared to other capillary networks, the glomerular capillary network is 100 times more permeable and has a higher hydrostatic pressure.

Q15:
A. F
B. T
C. T
D. F
E. F

The citric acid (Krebs) cycle occurs in the mitochondria of cells. Pyruvate (derived from glycolysis) is converted into acetyl-CoA, which enters the Krebs cycle by binding with oxaloacetate to form citrate. During the Krebs cycle, 2 molecules of carbon dioxide are produced per turn of the cycle. For each molecule of acetyl-CoA entering the cycle, 3 molecules of NADH are produced. The theoretical maximal yield of ATP through the oxidation of 1 molecule of glucose is 38 molecules of ATP, however this includes the steps of glycolysis, the Krebs cycle and oxidative phosphorylation.

Q16:
A. F
B. F
C. T
D. F
E. F

Only motilin out of the factors listed increases the rate of gastric emptying.

Q17:
A. T
B. F
C. T
D. T
E. F

The foetal circulation consists of a single umbilical vein which is relatively well oxygenated at 80% and two umbilical arteries (have a PaO_2 of 2.9kPa), which are derived from the iliac arteries and return blood to the placenta.

When blood enters the heart, the majority of the blood diverts across the foramen ovale to supply the systemic circulation. A small proportion of the blood flow goes to the lungs where the pulmonary vascular resistance is relatively high.

The brain has a relatively large oxygen extraction ratio so blood oxygen saturations in the superior vena cava are approximately 25%.

Q18:
A. T
B. F
C. T
D. T
E. T

Thyroid cells take up iodide via an ATP dependant process, that concentrates iodide in the thyroid gland. This is undertaken by the sodium-iodide pump.

Iodide and thyroglobulin (which is a large glycoprotein manufactured in the thyroid cells) are then moved into the thyroid colloid. In the thyroid colloid (not the thyroid cells), the iodide is converted into iodine (under the influence of thyroid peroxidase) and attached to the thyroglobulin molecule. The thyroglobulin molecule then splits into mono and di-iodothyronine molecules, which under the influence of thyroid peroxidase, form either tetra-iodothyronine, tri-iodothyronine or reverse tri-iodothyronine. Reverse tri-iodothyronine has no activity in the body as this isomer is unable to bind to thyroid receptors expressed in the body.

Q19:
A. T
B. F
C. F
D. F
E. T

Pancreatic fluid has a pH of 8 and is used to buffer the acidic contents leaving the stomach. Approximately 1500ml of pancreatic fluid is produced daily and its production is under the influence of numerous hormones, including secretin. Secretin increases the volume of pancreatic fluid produced and changes the composition of the fluid by increasing the bicarbonate concentration and decreasing the chloride concentration.

Pancreatic fluid contains numerous enzymes that are initially excreted as proenzymes, before being cleaved to active enzymes in the small bowel. An example of this is the secretion of trypsinogen by the acini cells which is then converted to the active trypsin in the duodenum under the influence of enteropeptidase.

The water and bicarbonate content of pancreatic fluid is entirely derived from the epithelial cells of the pancreatic duct.

Q20:
A. F
B. F
C. T
D. F
E. T

Myocardial contractility is increased by sympathetic stimulation, parasympathetic inhibition, increasing calcium ion concentration and inotropic agents. Contractility is decreased by hypoxia, acidosis, ischaemia and impaired atrioventricular coupling.

Questions 21-40

Q21:

Regarding the borders of the antecubital fossa:

A. The inferomedial border is formed by brachioradialis
B. The inferolateral border is formed by pronator teres
C. The floor of the antecubital fossa is formed by brachialis and supinator
D. The roof of the antecubital fossa is the deep fascia of the bicipital aponeurosis
E. The superior border is a line between the lateral and medial epicondyles of the humerus

Q22:

Regarding differences in the apex and base of the lung in a standing patient:

A. The ventilation perfusion ratio is higher at the base than apex
B. Ventilation is higher at the base of the lung than the apex
C. Blood flow is higher at the base of the lung than the apex
D. The apex of the lung is more acidotic than the base
E. Alveolar carbon dioxide partial pressure is the same at the apex and the base

Q23:

Regarding the comparison between cerebrospinal fluid (CSF) and plasma:

A. They have the same osmolality
B. CSF is more acidic than plasma
C. CSF has a higher concentration of glucose than plasma
D. CSF has a higher concentration of protein than plasma
E. CSF has a higher concentration of potassium than plasma

Q24:
Regarding renal clearance and renal blood flow:
A. Inulin is an appropriate agent to calculate renal clearance
B. If renal plasma flow and haematocrit are known, then renal blood flow can be calculated
C. Para-aminohippuric acid (PAH) is secreted by the proximal tubules
D. Inulin is freely filtered by the glomerulus
E. Para-aminohippuric acid (PAH) is unable to be filtered by the glomerulus

Q25:
Renal changes of pregnancy include:
A. Increased renal plasma flow
B. Increased glomerular filtration rate
C. Increased renal tubular reabsorption
D. Increased plasma urea concentration
E. Increased production of urine

Q26:
Regarding the adrenal cortex:
A. The zona glomerulosa secretes aldosterone
B. The zona fasicularis secretes cortisol
C. The zona reticularis secretes dehydroepiandrosterone
D. The zona glomerulosa secretes renin
E. The zona glomerulosa lies deep to the zona fasicularis

Q27:
Regarding the central nervous system:
A. Contains 150ml of cerebrospinal fluid
B. Cerebrospinal fluid travels from the lateral ventricles to the third ventricle via the foramina of Munro
C. Cerebrospinal fluid exits the fourth ventricle via the foramina of Lushka and the foramina of Magendie
D. The spinal cord contains 30 paired nerves
E. The spinal cord is approximately 90cm in length

Q28:

Regarding glycolysis (Embden-Myerhof pathway):

A. Consumes 2 molecules of ATP per molecule of glucose utilised
B. Generates 2 molecules of NADH per molecule of glucose utilised
C. Can only occur under aerobic conditions
D. Occurs in the mitochondria of cells
E. Ultimately creates pyruvate, which can then form acteyl-CoA to enter the citric acid (Kreb) cycle

Q29:

Regarding the synthesis of adrenaline (epinephrine):

A. Hydroxylation of phenylalanine creates tyrosine
B. N-methyltransferase converts adrenaline into noradrenaline
C. Decarboxylation of dopa forms dopamine
D. Adrenaline synthesis occurs in the adrenal medulla
E. Chromaffin cells produce adrenaline and noradrenaline

Q30:

Regarding the control of heart rate:

A. Parasympathetic innervation to the heart is from the left and right vagus nerves
B. Sympathetic innervation to the heart is derived from C5-T1 nerve fibres
C. Activation of the Bainbridge reflex leads to a slowing of the heart rate
D. Stimulation of the baroreceptor reflex by hypertension leads to a slowing of the heart rate
E. Activation of the lung volume stretch reflex leads to an increase in heart rate

Q31:
Regarding the brachial plexus:
A. It consists of 5 roots
B. It consists of 3 trunks
C. Each trunk divides into anterior and posterior divisions
D. The cords are named according to their position relative to the axillary vein
E. The supraclavicular nerve is derived from this plexus

Q32:
Regarding West's zones of the lung in an upright subject:
A. In zone 1, alveolar partial pressure is greater than arterial pressure
B. In zone 3, alveolar partial pressure is greater than venous and arterial pressure
C. In zone 2; arterial, venous pressure and alveolar partial pressures are equal
D. In zone 3, alveolar partial pressure is greater than venous pressure
E. Arterial pressure is always greater than venous pressure in zones 1,2 and 3

Q33:
Regarding the management of glucose by the kidney:
A. In health, glucose is not normally filtered by the glomerulus
B. Glucose is predominately reabsorbed in the distal nephron
C. Glucose is reabsorbed in combination with sodium
D. The inability to resorb glucose can lead to diuresis
E. The maximal rate of glucose reabsorption is $380mgmin^{-1}$

Q34:
Phase I reactions in hepatocytes include:
A. Dealkylation
B. Hydrolysis
C. Oxidation
D. Reduction
E. Sulphation

Q35:
Regarding erythrocytes and haemoglobin:
A. The average life span of an erythrocyte is 12 days
B. One haemoglobin A molecule consist of four polypeptide chains
C. The α peptide of haemoglobin is encoded on chromosome 15
D. Oxygenated haemoglobin exists in the taut configuration
E. Due to the absence of mitochondria, erythrocytes rely solely on glycolysis for energy production

Q36:
Regarding carbohydrate absorption:
A. The small bowel can only absorb glucose, fructose and galactose
B. Cellulose is broken down by pancreatic amylase
C. Absorption of glucose is an ATP dependant process
D. Galactose is absorbed via facilitated diffusion
E. Polysaccharides with a β linkage cannot be absorbed by the human body

Q37:
Regarding the classical coagulation cascade:
A. The extrinsic system is activated via tissue factor
B. Factor VIIa is required in the cleavage of factor X to factor Xa
C. The prothrombin time tests the integrity of the intrinsic pathway
D. The intrinsic pathway requires factor VIIIa as a cofactor to activate factor Xa
E. The final common pathway requires factor Va to change prothrombin to thrombin

Q38:
Regarding the comparison of type I and type II muscle fibres:
A. Type I fibres have more mitochondria than type II fibres
B. Type I fibres are quick to fatigue compared to type II fibres
C. Type I fibres have a high glycogen content relative to type II fibres
D. Type I fibres are fast to contract relative to type II fibres
E. Type I fibres rely on glycolysis, unlike type II fibres which rely on oxidative phosphorylation

Q39:

Regarding the eye:

A. Rod cells contain the pigment rhodopsin
B. Cone cells are responsible for colour vision
C. Rod cells are concentrated around the fovea
D. Normal intra-ocular pressure is 10-25mmHg
E. Aqueous humour is formed at a rate of 2mlmin^{-1}

Q40:

Regarding auscultation of the heart:

A. A split S1 sound is due to the closure of the tricuspid valve before the mitral valve
B. A loud S2 sound occurs when aortic or pulmonary diastolic pressure is elevated
C. A split S2 sound occurs when the aortic and pulmonary valves open asynchronously
D. S3 is classically heard in a dilated and non-compliant ventricle
E. S4 corresponds to the "c" wave of the central venous waveform

Q21:

A. F
B. F
C. T
D. T
E. T

Border	Structure
Inferomedial	Pronator teres
Inferolateral	Brachioradialis
Superior	Line between the lateral and medial epicondyles of the humerus
Floor	Supinator and brachialis
Roof	Deep fascia of the bicipital aponeurosis

Q22:

A. F
B. T
C. T
D. F
E. F

Both blood flow and lung ventilation are highest at the base of the lung, compared to the apex in the upright patient. However, blood flow falls faster than ventilation as you progress further up the lung towards the apex. This relative difference in the fall of these parameters leads to a change in the ventilation-perfusion relationship.

At the base, the ventilation-perfusion ratio is relatively small, but at the apex this ratio is relatively high.

In addition, the apex of the lung is more alkalotic than the base and the partial pressure of carbon dioxide is lower in the apex than the base.

Q23:
A. T
B. T
C. F
D. F
E. F

Cerebrospinal fluid (CSF) has the same osmolality as plasma at $290mOsmkg^{-1}H_2O$.

CSF usually contains:
- $0.3 gl^{-1}$ protein, which is far less than the protein content of plasma
- $4.8mmoll^{-1}$ glucose, which is less than the glucose concentration in plasma
- $147mmoll^{-1}$ sodium, which is similar to the concentration of sodium in plasma
- $2.9mmoll^{-1}$ potassium, which is less than the potassium concentration in plasma

The pH in the CSF is 7.32, which is slightly lower than plasma pH.

Q24:

A. T

B. T

C. T

D. T

E. F

Renal clearance is the volume of plasma that is cleared of a particular substance by the kidneys per unit time, as such it normally has the units of mlmin^{-1}. To calculate renal clearance you need an agent that is freely filtered at the glomerulus but is not secreted, reabsorbed, metabolised or synthesised by the kidney. An agent commonly used for this purpose is inulin.

The clearance of a substance by the kidney can be calculated by the following equation:

$$C_x = \frac{U_x V}{P_x}$$

C_x = Clearance of agent X

U_x = Urine concentration of agent X

V = Urine flow

P_x = Plasma concentration of agent X

If renal plasma flow and haematocrit are known, then the renal blood flow can be calculated from the following equation:

$$RBF = \frac{RPF \times 100}{Hct}$$

RBF = Renal blood flow

RPF = Renal plasma flow

Hct = Haematocrit

Para-aminohippuric acid (PAH) is used to calculate renal plasma flow as it is entirely removed from the plasma by the kidney through a combination of filtration and tubular secretion. The following equation can be utilised to calculate renal plasma flow:

$$RPF = \frac{U_{PAH}\ V}{P_{PAH}}$$

RPF = Renal plasma flow
U_{PAH} = Urine concentration of PAH
V = Urine flow
P_{PAH} = Plasma concentration of PAH

Q25:
A. T
B. T
C. F
D. F
E. T

Renal changes of pregnancy include an increase in renal plasma flow, glomerular filtration rate, urine volume and creatinine clearance. The plasma urea decreases as does the renal tubular reabsorption rate.

Q26:
A. T
B. T
C. T
D. F
E. F

The adrenal cortex contains three distinct layers, which synthesise and secrete different hormones. The zona glomerulosa (most superficial layer) secretes aldosterone, the zona fasicularis (intermediate layer) secretes cortisol and the zona reticularis secretes dehydroepiandrosterone (DHEA).

Renin is secreted by the juxtaglomerular cells of the kidney.

Q27:
A. T
B. T
C. T
D. F
E. F

The human adult spinal cord is approximately 45cm long and consists of 31 paired spinal nerves (8 cervical, 12 thoracic, 5 lumbar, 5 sacral and 1 coccygeal). Cerebrospinal fluid (CSF) is produced in the choroid plexus of the lateral ventricles and enters the third ventricle via the foramen of Munro. The CSF exits the fourth ventricle via the foramina of Lushka and the foramina of Magendie. Total CSF volume is around 150ml.

Q28:
A. T
B. T
C. F
D. F
E. T

Glycolysis (Embden-Myerhof pathway) occurs in the cytosol of cells in both aerobic and anaerobic conditions. It creates 2 molecules of pyruvate from a single molecule of glucose which can then be used to form acetyl-CoA to enter the Kreb's cycle.
In aerobic conditions, glycolysis requires 2 molecules of ATP per mole of glucose utilised and produces 4 molecules of ATP and 2

molecules of NADH, hence making an overall positive contribution to energy production.

Q29:
A. T
B. F
C. T
D. T
E. T

Adrenaline (epinephrine) synthesis requires the conversion of phenylalanine to tyrosine under the influence of hydroxylase. Tyrosine is then converted into dopa after further hydroxylation. Dopa is converted into dopamine via decarboxylation, which then undergoes further hydroxylation to form noradrenaline. Finally, adrenaline is formed by the enzyme N-methyltransferase's action on noradrenaline.

Chromaffin cells are capable of producing noradrenaline and adrenaline and these cells are predominately found in the adrenal medulla.

Q30:
A. T
B. F
C. F
D. T
E. T

The left vagus nerve supplies parasympathetic innervation to the sinoatrial node and the right vagus nerve supplies parasympathetic innervation to the atrial-ventricular node. Sympathetic innervation for the heart is derived from T1-T5 sympathetic fibres.

The Bainbridge reflex is a tachycardia due to increased atrial stretch. Stretching of the lung parenchyma also leads to a tachycardia.

Stimulation of baroreceptors due to hypertension leads to a bradycardia.

Q31:
A. T
B. T
C. T
D. F
E. F

The brachial plexus is derived from C5 to T1. It initially forms 5 roots, then 3 trunks (upper, middle and lower), followed by 6 divisions which then forms 3 cords (lateral, medial and posterior). The cords are named according to their position relative to the axillary artery. The supraclavicular nerve is formed from the cervical plexus.

Q32:
A. T
B. F
C. F
D. F
E. T

West's zones is a theoretical model of how the partial pressure of the alveolus, venous pressure and arterial pressure are related in three regions of the upright lung.
In zone 1 (at the apex): alveolar partial pressure is greater than arterial pressure which is greater than venous pressure.
In zone 2 (mid zone): arterial pressure is greater than alveolar partial pressure which is greater than venous pressure.
In zone 3 (at the base): arterial pressure is greater than venous pressure which is greater than alveolar partial pressure.

At no point in this model is venous pressure greater than arterial pressure.

Q33:
A. F
B. F
C. T
D. T
E. T

Glucose is a small, uncharged molecule that is able to pass freely through the glomerulus. In the nephron, the majority of glucose is reabsorbed in the proximal tubule, though it can also be reabsorbed in the distal nephron.

Reabsorption of glucose depends on a co-transport mechanism with sodium down sodium's electrochemical gradient. Provided that tubular glucose concentration does not exceed the reabsorption capacity of the kidney (around 380mgmin^{-1}), glyosuria should not occur. In reality, glycosuria only occurs in diseased states such as diabetes mellitus.

The inability to reabsorb glucose can lead to an osmotic diuresis.

Q34:
A. T
B. T
C. T
D. T
E. F

Phase I reactions in hepatocytes include: dealkylation, hydrolysis, oxidation and reduction.

Phase II reactions in hepatocytes include: sulphation, glucuronidation and acetylation.

Q35:
A. F
B. T
C. F
D. F
E. T

Erythrocytes contain no mitochondria or cell nucleus. They are dependant on glycolysis for energy production and have a life span of approximately 120 days.

Adult haemoglobin molecules are composed of 4 polypeptide chains. This quaternary structure comprises two α and two β peptides. The α chain is encoded on chromosome 16 and the β chain is encoded on chromosome 11.

As oxygen binds to haemoglobin, the conformation shifts from the taut state to the relaxed state.

Q36:
A. T
B. F
C. T
D. F
E. T

The body has to breakdown complex sugar molecules via enzymes in the small bowel before they can be absorbed. In humans, only glucose, fructose and galactose molecules can be absorbed by the brush border of the small bowel.

Glucose and galactose are absorbed via protein channels that utilise ATP and fructose absorption is via facilitated diffusion. Cellulose is a complex polysaccharide with β linkage between molecules. The body does not possess the enzymes required for its breakdown, therefore, cellulose cannot be absorbed by the body.

Q37:
A. T
B. T
C. F
D. T
E. T

The classical coagulation cascade is divided into the intrinsic and extrinsic pathway.

The extrinsic pathway is activated by the exposure of factor VII to tissue factor, resulting in the formation of factor VIIa. Factor VIIa then acts as a cofactor in the conversion factor X into factor Xa. The extrinsic pathway's function can be assessed with the prothrombin time assay.

The intrinsic pathway is activated by the exposure of factors XII and XI to substances found in the plasma. This ultimately causes factor IX to become factor IXa, which is essential for up regulating factor VIIIa. Factor VIIIa then changes factor X to factor Xa. The intrinsic pathway can be monitored with the activated partial thromboplastin time.

Once factor Xa is activated through either the intrinsic or extrinsic pathway, the final common pathway starts. Factor Xa activates factor V which then allows the transformation of prothrombin to thrombin. Thrombin then alters fibrinogen into fibrin which is able to form a stable clot.

Q38:

A. T
B. F
C. F
D. F
E. F

Type I muscle fibres are red in colour due to their relatively high mitochondrial content. They are slow to fatigue, rely mainly on oxidative phosphorylation and are capable of a sustained work rate without having to convert to anaerobic metabolism.

Type II muscle fibres fatigue quickly, have fewer mitochondria and have a higher glycogen content. They are quicker to respond to nerve impulses than type I fibres but incur an oxygen debt quicker.

Q39:

A. T
B. T
C. F
D. T
E. T

The eye contains two main types of cell that are responsible for interpreting light signals. The rods, which contain the pigment rhodopsin, are widely spread throughout the retina and are responsible for interpreting monochromatic light. Cone cells are concentrated on the fovea and are responsible for colour vision. There are approximately twelve times as many rods as cone cells in the human eye.

Normal intra-oscular pressure is 10-25mmHg and the aqueous humour is formed at a rate of 2mlmin^{-1}.

Q40:
A. F
B. T
C. F
D. T
E. F

The S1 sound corresponds to closure of the mitral and tricuspid valves and asynchronous closure of these valves leads to a split S1 sound. In normal physiological circumstances, the mitral valve closes 10ms earlier than the tricuspid valve, leading to the split S1 phenomena.

A loud S2 sound is heard when either the pulmonary or aortic pressure is raised. The S2 sound is split when the aortic and pulmonary valves close asynchronously.

S3 is a pathological sound that is associated with a dilated and non-compliant ventricle.

S4 is a pathological sound due to increased forcefulness of atrial contraction and would correspond to the "a" wave on the central venous waveform.

Questions 41-60

Q41:
The sciatic nerve:
A. Is derived from the L1 to L5 nerve roots
B. Passes through the greater sciatic foramen
C. Lies anterior to the acetabulum
D. Divides into the common peroneal nerve and tibial nerve
E. Forms the obturator nerve as it exits the pelvis

Q42:
The following are causes of physiological shunt:
A. The draining of coronary venous blood via the thebesian veins into the left ventricle
B. The draining of bronchial artery blood into the pulmonary veins
C. The reversal of blood flow across a ventricular septal defect with exercise
D. A patent ductus arteriosus in a 2 month old baby
E. Ebstein's anomaly

Q43:
Renin:
A. Is stored in the granular cells of the juxtaglomerular apparatus
B. Is released in response to parasympathetic stimulation
C. Is released when renal perfusion pressure decreases
D. Is released in response to a reduced sodium load being presented to the macula densa
E. Coverts angiotensin I to angiotensin II

Q44:
Regarding oxidative phosphorylation:
A. Occurs only in the mitochondria
B. Generates GTP
C. Cyanide is able to inhibit the electron transport chain
D. Chemiosmosis correctly describes the process of hydrogen ions moving down an electrochemical gradient during this process
E. Coenzyme Q_{10} is vital to the electron transfer chain process

Q45:
Regarding calcium homeostasis:
A. Calcium absorption mainly occurs in the terminal ileum
B. 1,25 dihydroxycholecalciferol increases calcium absorption from the intestine
C. Parathyroid hormone mobilises bone calcium stores
D. Calcitonin is produced by C (parafollicular) cells
E. Parathyroid hormone increases both calcium and phosphate plasma concentrations

Q46:
Respiratory changes at term in pregnancy compared to the non-pregnant state include:
A. An increase in tidal volume of 45%
B. An increase in residual volume of 20%
C. An increase in dead space of 45%
D. An increase in expiratory reserve volume of 25%
E. An increase in functional residual capacity of 30%

Q47:

The following are essential amino acids:

A. Alanine
B. Aspartic acid
C. Leucine
D. Methionine
E. Valine

Q48:

Regarding adrenergic receptors:

A. They are G protein coupled receptors
B. Stimulation of α_1 receptors induces smooth muscle contraction
C. Stimulation of β_1 receptors decreases renin secretion
D. Stimulation of β_2 receptors induces bronchial smooth muscle relaxation
E. Stimulation of β_3 receptors induces lipolysis in adipose tissue

Q49:

The median nerve innervates the following muscles:

A. Flexor carpi radialis
B. Flexor carpi ulnaris
C. Flexor digitorum superficialis
D. Palmaris longus
E. Pronator teres

Q50:

The following values are correct for a 70kg male at rest:

A. Cardiac output 4.5lmin^{-1}
B. Cardiac index 300mlmin^{-1}m^{-2}
C. Systemic vascular resistance 2000dyn.s.cm^{-5}
D. Stroke index 70mlm^{-2}
E. Pulmonary vascular resistance 200dyn.s.cm^{-5}

Q51:

The following structures traverse the superior orbital fissure:

A. Inferior branch of the oculomotor nerve
B. Inferior ophthalmic vein
C. Lacrimal nerve
D. Nasociliary nerve
E. Optic nerve

Q52:

Regarding the concept of work of breathing:

A. Lung efficiency is approximately 30%
B. At rest, the lung consumes approximately 20% of total body oxygen supply
C. During hyperventilation, the lung consumes approximately 40% of total body oxygen supply
D. Work against the elastic recoil of the lung is stored as potential energy
E. Joules are appropriate units for the work of breathing per second

Q53:

Angiotensin II:

A. Stimulates the release of aldosterone
B. Acts as a systemic vasoconstrictor
C. Stimulates the release of renin
D. Leads to increased sodium reabsorption from the kidney
E. Stimulates water retention

Q54:
Regarding the distribution of blood flow at rest and during exercise:
A. Blood flow to the brain is constant during exercise and rest
B. Skeletal muscle blood flow increases 10 fold during exercise compared to rest
C. Blood flow to the kidneys is constant during exercise and rest
D. Coronary artery blood flow does not increase during exercise
E. Blood flow to the abdominal viscera decreases during exercise

Q55:
Regarding the absorption of iron:
A. Can be absorbed as either haem or free iron
B. Is primarily absorbed in the terminal ileum
C. Iron absorption is modulated by intrinsic factor
D. Iron binds intracellularly with apoferritin to from ferritin
E. The vast majority of iron is absorbed by the intestine

Q56:
Regarding the gamma aminobutyric acid type A (GABA$_A$) receptor:
A. It is a metabotropic receptor
B. When activated enables the uptake of chloride ions into the cell
C. Has an inhibitory role in the central nervous system
D. Has a pentameric structure
E. Has separate binding sites for GABA and benzodiazepines

Q57:
The following are descending tracts of the spinal cord:
A. Corticospinal tract
B. Gracile and cuneate tracts
C. Recticulospinal tract
D. Rubrospinal tract
E. Spinothalamic tract

Q58:

The following statements are true concerning plasma and intracellular fluid:

A. Plasma has a higher concentration of calcium than intracellular fluid

B. Plasma has a higher concentration of magnesium than intracellular fluid

C. Plasma has a higher concentration of sodium than intracellular fluid

D. Plasma has a higher concentration of potassium than intracellular fluid

E. Plasma has a higher concentration of protein than intracellular fluid

Q59:

Regarding immunoglobulin (antibody):

A. Produced by plasma cells

B. Have a specific antigen binding site

C. Are able to undergo class switching

D. There are 4 isotopes of immunoglobulin in humans

E. Consist of 1 heavy and 1 light chain

Q60:

Regarding the cardiac action potential:

A. The resting membrane potential is -60mV

B. During phase 0, fast sodium channels open and potassium channels close

C. During phase 1, the membrane potential goes from +20mV to 0mV

D. Phase 2 requires the continued influx of calcium ions via T-type channels

E. During phase 3, rapid depolarisation occurs due to potassium efflux

Answers 41-60

Q41:
A. F
B. T
C. F
D. T
E. F

The sciatic nerve is the longest nerve in the human body and is derived from the L1 to S3 nerve roots. The sciatic nerve exits via the greater sciatic foramen and lies posterior to the acetabulum. It divides into the common peroneal and tibial nerves. The obturator nerve is formed from the lumbar plexus, not the sciatic nerve.

Q42:
A. T
B. T
C. F
D. F
E. F

Shunt is the movement of blood into the arterial circulation, without it moving through ventilated areas of lung. Shunt can either be physiological (i.e. normal) or pathological. The 2 causes of physiological shunt in adults are drainage of coronary artery blood directly into the left ventricle via the thebesian veins and the drainage of bronchial artery blood into the pulmonary veins. Physiological shunt accounts for approximately 2% of cardiac output.

Pathological causes of shunt include non-closure of a patent ductus arteriosus, right to left shunt due to a ventricular septal defect or atrial septal defect and certain eponymous conditions such as Epstein's anomaly.

Q43:
A. T
B. F
C. T
D. T
E. F

Renin is stored in the granular cells of the juxtaglomerular apparatus. Renin is released in response to reducing renal perfusion pressures, stimulation by the sympathetic nervous system or the macula densa being exposed to a low sodium load. Once released, renin acts to cleave angiotensin I from angiotensinogen.

Q44:
A. T
B. F
C. T
D. T
E. T

Oxidative phosphorylation takes place inside the mitochondria. It generates ATP via the movement of hydrogen ions down an electrochemical gradient (chemiosmosis).

Cyanide is able to inhibit the electron transport chain and Coenzyme Q_{10} is vital to the electron transfer chain process.

Q45:
A. F
B. T
C. T
D. T
E. F

Calcium homeostasis is under the influence of parathyroid hormone (PTH), vitamin D (and its derivatives) and calcitonin. PTH is secreted by chief cells in the parathyroid glands and causes an increase in calcium levels via the mobilisation of bone calcium, reabsorption of calcium in the distal tubule of the kidney and by increasing 1,25-dihydroxycholecalciferol levels. PTH secretions lead to a decrease in phosphate levels.

Calcium is mainly absorbed in the duodenum of the small bowel under the influence of 1,25-dihydroxycholecalciferol. 1,25-dihydroxycholecalciferol is derived from 25-hydroxycholecalciferol under the influence of an enzyme located in the kidney. 25-hydroxycholecalciferol is manufactured in the liver and its substrate is supplied from either the absorption of vitamin D3 in the gut or by the action of UV radiation on 7-dehydroxycholesterol to form cholecalciferol.

Calcitonin is produced by C (parafollicular) cells and works to reduce both phosphate and calcium levels in the body.

Q46:
A. T
B. F
C. T
D. F
E. F

Respiratory changes at term in pregnancy compared to the non-pregnant state include:
- tidal volume increases by 45%
- dead space increases by 45%
- residual volume decreases by 20%
- expiratory reserve volume decreases by 25%
- functional residual capacity decreases by 30%

Q47:

A. F
B. F
C. T
D. T
E. T

The following are the 9 essential amino acids: histidine, isoleucine, leucine, lysine, methionine, phenylalanine, threonine, tryptophan and valine. An essential amino acid is defined as an amino acid that cannot be manufactured by the body.

Q48:

A. T
B. T
C. F
D. T
E. T

Adrenergic receptors are G protein coupled receptors that have a large number of effects on the body.

Stimulation of the α_1 receptors induces smooth muscle contraction in the ureters, vas deferens, hair, uterus, bronchial walls and blood vessels.

Stimulation of β_1 receptors increases renin secretion and cardiac output (through positive inotropic, dromotropic and inotropic effects).

Stimulation of β_2 receptors induces smooth muscle relaxation in the bronchi, uterus and gut. It also stimulates glycogenolysis and gluconeogenesis.

Stimulation of β_3 receptors induces lipolysis in adipose tissue.

Q49:
A. T
B. F
C. T
D. T
E. T

The median nerve innervates all the flexor muscles of the forearm except flexor carpi ulnaris and part of flexor digitorum profundus, which are supplied by the ulnar nerve.

Q50:
A. T
B. F
C. F
D. F
E. T

Cardiac output for a 70kg man at rest is approximately 4.5lmin^{-1} with a cardiac index of $3 \text{lmin}^{-1}\text{m}^{-2}$ and a stroke index of $50\text{-}60 \text{mlm}^{-2}$. The systemic vascular resistance is $1000\text{-}1500 \text{dyn.s.cm}^{-5}$ and the pulmonary vascular resistance is 200dyn.s.cm^{-5}.

Q51:
A. T
B. F
C. T
D. T
E. F

The optic nerve and ophthalmic artery enter the orbit through the optic canal.

The inferior ophthalmic vein, infra-orbital artery and infra-orbital nerve enter the orbit through the inferior orbital fissure.

The superior orbital fissure contains the lacrimal nerve, frontal nerve, trochlear nerve, superior ophthalmic vein, oculomotor nerve (superior and inferior branches), nasociliary nerve and abducens nerve.

Q52:
A. F
B. F
C. F
D. T
E. F

The work of breathing is difficult to measure, but it is believed that the lungs are around 5-10% efficient. At rest (with shallow breathing) the lungs consume approximately 5% of total body oxygen and this increases to 30% with exercise.

Inspiration is an active process with some energy lost due to the resistive forces of the lung. However, the force used to overcome the elastic recoil properties of the lung is stored as potential energy which is then used during the passive expiratory phase.

Total work of breathing can be measured in joules, but work of breathing per second is measured in watts.

Q53:
A. T
B. T
C. F
D. T
E. T

Angiotensin II is an octapeptide, created through the conversion of angiotensin I to angiotensin II by angiotensin converting enzyme (ACE). Angiotensin I is formed from angiotensinogen (produced by the liver). The formation of angiotensin I is rate-limited by renin, a protease produced by the juxtaglomerular cells in the kidney. Angiotensin II inhibits renin secretion via a negative feedback loop. Angiotensin II is a potent vasoconstrictor that stimulates thirst, water reabsorption, sodium reabsorption and the release of aldosterone.

Q54:
A. T
B. T
C. F
D. F
E. T

Cardiac output increases threefold during exercise and the amount of blood flow to different organs changes considerably. Skeletal blood flow increases 10 fold from 1200mlmin^{-1} to over 12000mlmin^{-1}. Coronary artery blood flow increases from 250mlmin^{-1} to 750mlmin^{-1}. During exercise the amount of blood flow to the kidneys and abdominal viscera decreases but blood flow to the brain is maintained at 750mlmin^{-1}.

Q55:
A. T
B. F
C. F
D. T
E. F

Iron is absorbed from the duodenum and jejunum as either free iron or as part of a haem molecule. Normally, only a tiny proportion of the iron content of the bowel is taken up by the human body. Iron absorption is either via pinocytosis for haem species of iron or via active transport with a specific receptor. Once inside the cell, the iron binds to apoferritin thus forming ferritin. Iron is transported around the body bound to the transferrin molecule.

Intrinsic factor is secreted by parietal cells and is part of the mechanism of vitamin B_{12} absorption in the terminal ileum, it does not influence iron absorption.

Q56:
A. F
B. T
C. T
D. T
E. T

The gamma aminobutyric acid type A ($GABA_A$) receptor is an inotropic receptor which allows the passage of chloride down its concentration gradient when activated. This leads to hyper polarisation of the cell and a reduced ability to send action potentials.

The $GABA_A$ receptor comprises a pentameric structure with two GABA binding sites and a separate benzodiazepine binding site.

Q57:
A. T
B. F
C. T
D. T
E. F

The corticospinal, rubrospinal and recticulospinal tracts are descending pathways.

Q58:
A. T
B. F
C. T
D. F
E. F

Substance	Intracellular concentration (mmoll^{-1})	Plasma concentration (mmoll^{-1})
Calcium	1	2.7
Magnesium	40	1
Sodium	10	148
Potassium	159	4.3
Protein	45	15

Q59:
A. T
B. T
C. T
D. F
E. F

Immunoglobulin (antibody) is produced by B-cells and plasma cells (which are modified B-cells). There are 5 different isotopes of immunoglobulin (IgA, IgD, IgE, IgG and IgM), which can undergo class switching. An immunoglobulin molecule consists of 2 heavy and 2 light chains, they have a specific antigen binding site.

Q60:

A. F
B. T
C. T
D. F
E. T

The cardiac action potential consists of phases 0,1,2,3 and 4. Phase 0 occurs when the threshold potential is reached and fast sodium channels are opened, increasing the membrane potential to +20mV. During phase 1, a brief period of depolarisation to 0mV occurs due to the outflow of potassium from the cell. Phase 2 (plateau phase) corresponds to the opening of L-type calcium channels that maintain the action potential at around 0mV. Phase 3 is the rapid depolarisation phase due to the outflow of potassium, which returns the membrane potential to its resting potential of -90mV. During phase 4, an equilibrium between chemical and electrical forces is reached. Phase 0 will begin again when the threshold potential is reached.

Questions 61-80

Q61:

Regarding the borders of the inguinal canal:

A. The anterior boundary is formed by the aponeurosis of the external oblique muscle

B. The deep inguinal ring is an opening in the external oblique aponeurosis

C. The floor is formed by the inguinal ligament

D. The posterior boundary is formed by the conjoint tendon and fascia transversalis

E. The roof is formed by the transverse abdominis and internal oblique muscles

Q62:

Regarding the control of ventilation:

A. The dorsal respiratory group is mainly associated with expiration

B. The apneustic centre is contained in the lower pons

C. The pneumotaxic centre regulates inspiratory volume

D. The medullary respiratory centre is located beneath the floor of the third ventricle

E. Absence of the pneumotaxic centre is not compatible with life

Q63:

Regarding renal blood supply:

A. The kidneys receive 20-25% of cardiac output at rest

B. The inner medulla of the kidney receives a higher blood flow rate per unit mass than the outer medulla of the kidney

C. The renal artery branches into the arcuate arteries

D. The renal cortex of the kidney receives a higher blood flow rate per unit mass than the renal medulla

E. Interlobular arteries are derived from the arcuate arteries

Q64:

The following are polypeptide hormones:

A. Follicle stimulating hormone
B. Insulin
C. Testosterone
D. Thyroid stimulating hormone
E. Vasopressin

Q65:

The following will increase cerebral blood flow:

A. Increasing the arterial partial pressure of carbon dioxide from 4kPa to 6kPa
B. Decreasing the arterial partial pressure of oxygen from 13kPa to 9kPa
C. Increasing cerebral metabolic rate from 3ml100g^{-1}min^{-1} to 6ml100g^{-1}min^{-1}
D. Increasing the systemic mean arterial pressure to 160mmHg in a normally normotensive individual
E. Decreasing the body's temperature by 5°C

Q66:

Regarding body water:

A. A 70kg man would be expected to have a total body water of 42L
B. A 70kg man would be expected to have an intracellular fluid volume of 14L
C. A 70kg man would be expected to have a plasma volume of 5L
D. A 70kg man would be expected to have an interstitial fluid volume of 11L
E. Total body water can be measured with radio labelled albumin

Q67:

The tibial nerve:

A. Is a branch of the femoral nerve
B. Supplies the gastrocnemius muscle
C. Supplies the flexor hallucis longus muscle
D. Divides into medial and lateral plantar nerves in the calf
E. Runs anterior to the medial malleolus

Q68:

The following are structures of the basal ganglia:

A. Caudate nucleus
B. Globus pallidus
C. Periaqueductal gray matter
D. Substantia nigra
E. Subthalamic nucleus

Q69:

The following amino acids can be utilised in gluconeogenesis to form glucose:

A. Alanine
B. Cysteine
C. Glycine
D. Leucine
E. Valine

Q70:

Regarding cardiac muscle cells:

A. Cardiac muscle is striated
B. The thick filaments are composed of myosin molecules
C. During systole, the calcium ion concentration increases 100 fold
D. Calcium binds to tropomyosin, allowing the actin and myosin to interact
E. Calcium is stored in the sarcoplasmic reticulum

Q71:
Regarding the first rib:

A. The scalenus medius muscle inserts onto the first rib
B. The subclavian artery travels inferior to the first rib in the subclavian groove
C. Serratus anterior attaches to the first rib on the inner medial curve
D. The subclavian vein is anterior to the subclavian artery
E. Has a tubercle for the attachment of scalenus anterior

Q72:
Regarding physiological adaption to high altitude:

A. Hyperventilation due to hypoxia occurs
B. Renal bicarbonate excretion is reduced
C. Polycythaemia occurs and blood viscosity increases
D. Pulmonary arterial pressure increases
E. 2,3-diphosphoglycerate concentrations decrease

Q73:
Regarding the loop of Henle:

A. Fluid entering the distal tubule after the loop of Henle is hypertonic
B. The thick ascending limb of the loop of Henle actively excretes ions
C. The ascending limb of the loop of Henle is permeable to water
D. 15% of nephrons in the kidney have long loops
E. Osmolality of tubular fluid in the renal cortex can reach 1400mOsmkg^{-1}H$_2$0

Q74:
The following are fat soluble vitamins:
A. Vitamin B1 (thiamine)
B. Vitamin B2 (riboflavin)
C. Vitamin B3 (niacin)
D. Vitamin B6 (pyridoxine)
E. Vitamin B12 (cyanocobalamin)

Q75:
Regarding intracranial contents and pressure:
A. Normal intracranial pressure is between 5 and 15cmH$_2$0
B. Cerebral perfusion pressure equals the mean arterial pressure minus the intracranial pressure
C. The Munro-Kellie doctrine links increasing cerebral perfusion pressure to increasing intracranial pressure
D. Normally the brain parenchyma comprises 85% of intracranial volume
E. Normally cerebrospinal fluid comprises 5% of intracranial volume

Q76:
IgG antibody:
A. Is the most common type of antibody found in the circulation
B. Forms an essential part of cell mediated immunity
C. Activates the classical pathway of the complement system
D. Is contained in colostrum
E. Is able to cross the placenta

Q77:

The following factors delay gastric emptying:

A. Distention of the stomach
B. Distention of the duodenum
C. Secretin
D. Pain
E. Sympathetic stimulation

Q78:

Regarding the larynx:

A. It has three paired cartilages
B. It has three unpaired cartilages
C. It has three extrinsic muscles
D. The cricothyroid muscle is supplied by the inferior laryngeal nerve
E. Venous supply to the larynx is from the superior and inferior thyroid veins

Q79:

Regarding the N-methyl-D-aspartate (NMDA) receptor:

A. It is an inotropic receptor
B. It has a glutamate binding site
C. Magnesium can prevent the passage of other cations through the central pore
D. It has a pentameric structure
E. Glycine is a co-agonist of this receptor

Q80:

The following pressures at rest in the cardiovascular system are correct:

A. Right atrial pressure of 4mmHg
B. Mean pulmonary artery wedge pressure of 20mmHg
C. Mean pulmonary artery pressure of 30mmHg
D. Left ventricular end diastolic pressure of 70mmHg
E. Left ventricular systolic pressure of 120mmHg

Answers 61-80

Q61:
A. T
B. F
C. T
D. T
E. T

Border	Structure
Anterior	Aponeurosis of the external oblique muscle
Posterior	Fascia transversalis and conjoint tendon (medial third)
Floor	Inguinal ligament
Roof	Transverse abdominis and internal oblique muscle
Deep inguinal ring	Opening in the fascia transversalis
Superficial inguinal ring	Opening in the external oblique aponeurosis

Q62:
A. F
B. T
C. T
D. F
E. F

The pneumotaxic centre is located in the upper pons and is responsible for inhibiting respiration, it therefore controls the volume of inspiration. It is not essential for life but works to fine tune the inspiratory effort.

The apneustic centre is located in the lower pons. It increases inspiratory effort and loss of this centre can lead to gasping.

The medullary respiratory group (MRG) is located in the reticular formation which is just below the fourth ventricle in the medulla. The MRG is responsible for the generation of respiratory rhythm.

The dorsal respiratory group is responsible for inspiration and the ventral inspiratory group is responsible for expiration.

Q63:
A. T
B. F
C. F
D. T
E. T

At rest, the kidneys receive approximately 20-25% of cardiac output. The renal arteries supply the vast majority of blood flow to the kidneys and they branch into the interlobar arteries. The interlobar arteries then branch into arcuate arteries which then branch into the interlobular arteries.

The inner medulla of the kidney receives $20\text{ml}100\text{g}^{-1}\text{min}^{-1}$ of blood compared to the outer medulla which receives $100\text{ml}100\text{g}^{-1}\text{min}^{-1}$ of blood.

The renal cortex receives $500\text{ml}100\text{g}^{-1}\text{min}^{-1}$ of blood, which is greater than the flow rate per unit mass to the renal medulla.

Q64:
A. F
B. T
C. F
D. F
E. T

Polypeptide hormones include: vasopressin, oxytocin, calcitonin, insulin and adrenocorticotrophic hormone.

Glycoprotein hormones include: follicle stimulating hormone, leuteinizing hormone and thyroid stimulating hormone.

Steroid hormones include: testosterone, oestrogen, aldosterone and corticosteroid.

Q65:
A. T
B. F
C. T
D. T
E. F

Cerebral blood flow is normally $50ml100g^{-1}min^{-1}$ but this can be altered by either:
- Increasing the partial pressure of carbon dioxide in the blood. This relationship is linear between 4-8kPa and tapers at the lower and higher ends of this range.
- Inducing significant hypoxia will increases cerebral blood flow, however the cerebral blood flow rate is remarkably linear down to arterial oxygen partial pressures of around 7kPa and then rapidly increases.
- Increasing the cerebral metabolic rate increases the cerebral blood flow rate in a linear fashion.

- Due to autoregulation the cerebral blood flow rate is able to maintain a constant flow rate between mean arterial pressures (MAP) of 50-150mmHg in normotensive individuals. However, MAP values greater than 150mmHg will increase cerebral blood flow rate and pressures below 50mmHg will reduce cerebral blood flow rate.
- Decreasing the patient's temperature will reduce cerebral metabolic activity, therefore it will indirectly reduce cerebral blood flow.

Q66:
A. T
B. F
C. F
D. T
E. F

Body compartment	Description and notes	Amount for a 70Kg man
Total body water	Usually 60% of body mass	42 litres
Intracellular fluid	2/3 of total body water	28 litres
Extracellular fluid	1/3 of total body water	14 litres
Plasma volume	blood volume - red cell volume	3 litres
Blood volume	plasma volume + red cell volume	5 litres
Interstitial volume	extracellular fluid - plasma volume	11 litres

Total body water can be measured using antipyrine D_2O.

Q67:
A. F
B. T
C. T
D. F
E. F

The tibial nerve is a branch of the sciatic nerve and is responsible for innervating the gastrocnemius, popliteus, tibias posterior and soleus muscles in the calf. The nerve travels with the tibial artery posterior to the medial malleolus and then divides into medial and lateral plantar nerves. In the foot, the nerve innervates the flexor hallucis longus and flexor digitorum longus muscles.

Q68:
A. T
B. T
C. F
D. T
E. T

The structures of the basal ganglia are the caudate nucleus, globus pallidus, substantial nigra, subthalamic nucleus and putamen.

The periaqueductal gray matter lies within the midbrain.

Q69:
A. T
B. T
C. T
D. F
E. T

Most amino acids can be utilised in gluconeogenesis to form glucose, however, leucine and lysine are ketogenic and not glucogenic.

Q70:
A. T
B. T
C. F
D. F
E. T

Cardiac muscle is striated and forms a functional syncytium with adjacent cells. During systole, calcium is released from the sarcoplasmic reticulum which increases intracellular calcium concentration by a factor of 1000. The calcium then binds to troponin which causes a conformational change in tropomyosin, allowing actin and myosin to bind. During diastole, the calcium ions are stored in the sarcoplasmic reticulum.

Q71:
A. T
B. F
C. F
D. T
E. T

The first rib is short and relatively flat compared to the other ribs. It has separate grooves for the subclavian artery and vein which cross the rib on its superior surface. The subclavian vein groove is anterior to the subclavian artery groove. The scalenus medius, scalenus anterior and serratus anterior muscles directly attach to the first rib.
The serratus anterior muscle attaches to the outer lateral surface of the rib, unlike scalenus anterior which attaches to a tubercle on the inner aspect of the rib.

Q72:
A. T
B. F
C. T
D. T
E. F

Physiological adaptions to altitude include:
- Increase in the minute ventilation due to hyperventilation which is stimulated by hypoxia.
- The increased minute ventilation initially causes a respiratory alkalosis which is altered over 2-3 days by the excretion of bicarbonate in the kidneys to normalise the pH.
- Polycythaemia occurs to optimise the oxygen carrying capacity of the blood, but this can lead to increased viscosity.
- Initially, 2-3diphosphoglycerate concentration increases as you ascend.
- Due to alveolar hypoxia, pulmonary vasoconstriction occurs, which increases right ventricular pressure and pulmonary artery pressure. This can cause right ventricular remodelling and strain.

Q73:
A. F
B. T
C. F
D. T
E. F

The loop of Henle acts to concentrate the interstitum of the inner medulla of the kidney. This is achieved by the extrusion of salt by the thick ascending limb and the impermeable nature of the ascending limb to water. This leads to a relative hypotonicity of the tubular fluid entering the distal nephron. Water is primarily removed by the collecting ducts under the influence of anti-diuretic hormone (vasopressin) and the osmotic gradient generated by the loop of Henle.

The tip of the loop of Henle in the inner medulla can reach osmolalities of around $1400mOsmkg^{-1}H_2O$, but in the cortex the osmolality is around $290mOsmkg^{-1}H_2O$.

Approximately 15% of the nephrons in the kidney are considered to have long loops of Henle.

Q74:
A. F
B. F
C. F
D. F
E. F

Vitamins A, D, E and K are considered fat soluble.

Q75:
A. F
B. T
C. F
D. T
E. T

Intracranial pressure is normally between 5 to 15mmHg.

Cerebral perfusion pressure equals the mean arterial pressure minus the intracranial pressure. However, if central venous pressure is greater than intracranial pressure the equation alters to cerebral perfusion pressure equaling mean arterial pressure minus central venous pressure.

The Munro-Kellie doctrine describes the pressure-volume relationship of the intracranial contents.

Normally, the brain parenchyma comprises 85% of intracranial volume, the cerebrospinal fluid 5% of intracranial volume and the blood 10% of intracranial volume.

Q76:
A. T
B. F
C. T
D. T
E. T

The IgG antibody plays an essential role in the humoral immunity pathway. It is able to activate the classical pathway of complement, cross the placenta, neutralise toxins, augment cell mediated cytotoxicity and directly initiate proteolyses. It is present in breast milk.

Q77:
A. F
B. T
C. T
D. T
E. T

Distention of the stomach and parasympathetic stimulation increase the rate of gastric emptying.

Duodenal distention, pain, anxiety, sympathetic stimulation and secretin delay the rate of gastric emptying.

Q78:
A. T
B. T
C. T
D. F
E. T

The larynx has three paired (arytenoid, corniculate and cuneiform cartilages) and three unpaired cartilages (epiglottis, thyroid and cricoid cartilages).

It has six intrinsic muscles (posterior cricoarytenoid, lateral cricoarytenoid, interarytenoid, thyroarytenoid, vocalis and cricothyroid muscles) and three extrinsic muscles (sternothyroid, thyrohyoid and inferior constrictor muscles).

The cricothyroid muscle is the only intrinsic muscle supplied by the superior laryngeal nerve, all the others are supplied by the inferior (recurrent) laryngeal nerve.

Arterial supply to the larynx is from the superior and inferior laryngeal arteries and venous drainage is from the superior and inferior thyroid veins.

Q79:
A. T
B. T
C. T
D. F
E. T

The N-methyl-D-aspartate (NMDA) receptor has a heterotetramer structure comprising two GluN1 and two GLuN2 subunits and acts as an inotropic receptor. It has binding sites for glutamate and its coenzyme, glycine, which when activated together increase the efficiency of cation movement across the membrane. Whilst the central pore of the channel will allow passage of any cation, the main cation that is moved by this receptor is calcium. Magnesium can inhibit the transmission of other cations across the membrane.

Q80:
A. T
B. F
C. F
D. F
E. T

Right atrial pressure is the same as the mean central venous pressure at approximately 4mmHg (range 0-8mmHg). Mean pulmonary artery wedge pressure is around 10mmHg (range 5-15mmHg) and the mean pulmonary artery pressure is 15mmHg (range 10-20mmHg). Left ventricular end diastolic pressure is 7mmHg (range 4-12mmHg) with the left ventricular systolic pressure being 120mmHg (range 90-140mmHg).

Questions 81-100

Q81:
Regarding the vagus nerve:
A. Exits the skull through the jugular foramen
B. Descends through the neck in the carotid sheath
C. The right vagus nerve travels posterior to the right subclavian artery
D. The left vagus nerve travels posterior to the left brachiocephalic vein
E. Supplies motor innervation to the diaphragm

Q82:
Regarding lung volumes:
A. Total lung capacity equals the residual volume plus the vital capacity
B. Functional residual capacity equals the residual volume plus the expiratory reserve volume
C. Inspiratory reserve volume equals the tidal volume plus the inspiratory capacity
D. Closing volume is always less than residual capacity
E. Inspiratory and expiratory reserve volumes are equal

Q83:
Regarding the stomach:
A. Approximately 2000ml of gastric juice is produced per day
B. Chief cells secrete pepsinogen
C. Parietal cells (oxyntic) cells secrete gastrin
D. Histamine stimulates gastric acid secretion
E. The gastric mucosa is covered by a 6mm layer of mucus

Q84:

Regarding thyroid hormone:

A. The majority of thyroid hormone secreted is in the form of tri-iodothyronine
B. Tri-iodothyronine is more potent than tetra-iodothyronine
C. Albumin has the greatest capacity for binding thyroid hormone
D. 10% of thyroid hormone circulates in an unbound manner
E. The liver and kidney are capable of de-iodinating thyroid hormone

Q85:

Cardiovascular changes at term in pregnancy compared to the non-pregnant state include:

A. An increase in cardiac output of 50%
B. An increase in heart rate of 25%
C. An increase in systemic vascular resistance of 20%
D. An increase in pulmonary vascular resistance of 30%
E. An increase in left ventricular end diastolic volume of 10%

Q86:

Regarding biliary secretion:

A. The gallbladder can store approximately 60ml of bile
B. Approximately 1000ml of bile is produced daily
C. Bile salts are necessary for the absorption of water soluble vitamins
D. Bile has a pH of 4-5
E. More than 90% of bile salts are reabsorbed and re-used from the small intestine

Q87:

The following vitamin deficiencies are correctly paired to their resulting diseases:

A. Thiamine deficiency and beriberi
B. Vitamin B1 deficiency and Wernicke-Korsakoff syndrome
C. Vitamin A deficiency and xerophthalmia
D. Vitamin D deficiency and rickets
E. Vitamin B12 deficiency and pernicious anaemia

Q88:

Regarding the blood supply to the brain:

A. The brain receives 15% of cardiac output at rest
B. The vertebral arteries are derived from the common carotid arteries
C. The basilar artery is formed by the fusion of the vertebral arteries
D. The basilar artery travels on the ventral aspect of the pons
E. The middle cerebral artery supplies the majority of the corpus callosum

Q89:

The following are examples of Type IV hypersensitivity reactions:

A. Mantoux test
B. Contact dermatitis
C. Rheumatic heart disease
D. Chronic transplant rejection
E. Anaphylaxis

Q90:

Regarding prostaglandins:

A. Every prostaglandin contains 20 carbon atoms
B. They bind to G protein coupled receptors
C. $PGF_{2\alpha}$ is associated with uterine relaxation
D. $PGF_{2\alpha}$ is associated with bronchoconstriction
E. Arachidonic acid can be manufactured from phospholipid and diacylglycerol

Q91:

Regarding the major histocompatibility complex (MHC):

A. Enables antibody presentation for the triggering of T cell responses
B. All nucleated cells in the body express MHC class 1 molecules
C. Dendritic cells, B cells and macrophages present antigens to T helper cells
D. MHC gene expression is co-dominant
E. Forms an essential part of humoral immunity

Q92:

Regarding the radial nerve:

A. Is derived from the medial cord of the brachial plexus
B. Is formed from the nerve roots C5, C6 and C7
C. Innervates the triceps brachii muscle
D. Innervates extensor carpi ulnaris
E. Radial nerve injury may present with wrist drop

Q93:

Regarding the partial pressures of gasses between the mother and foetus:

A. The maternal arterial system has a higher partial pressure of oxygen than the foetal umbilical vein
B. The foetal umbilical vein has a higher partial pressure of carbon dioxide than the umbilical arteries
C. The foetal umbilical arteries have a higher partial pressure of oxygen than the umbilical vein
D. The maternal arterial system has a higher partial pressure of carbon dioxide than the foetal umbilical vein
E. The maternal arterial system has a higher partial pressure of carbon dioxide than the foetal umbilical arteries

Q94:

Regarding inhibitors of coagulation:

A. Protein C is a vitamin K dependant factor
B. Protein C is activated by the thrombomodulin-thrombin complex
C. Protein C and protein S act together to inhibit factor Va and factor VIIa
D. Plasminogen directly breaks down fibrin
E. Tranexamic acid and aprotinin can inhibit the activity of plasmin

Q95:

Mechanisms of placental transport include:

A. Simple diffusion
B. Facilitated diffusion
C. Secondary active transport
D. Active transport
E. Pinocytosis

Q96:

The following hormones are contained in the anterior lobe of the pituitary gland:

A. Follicle stimulating hormone
B. Growth hormone
C. Oxytocin
D. Thyrotropin releasing hormone
E. Vasopressin

Q97:

Regarding the vomiting process:

A. Afferent nerve fibres involved in vomiting are derived from the vagus nerve
B. Mechano and chemo receptors in the gut can stimulate the vomiting reflex
C. The chemoreceptor trigger zone is located in the pineal body of the brain
D. The chemoreceptor trigger zone only expresses muscarinic receptors
E. The efferent nerve fibres involved in vomiting are derived from the vagus nerve

Q98:

The following conditions increase a person's functional residual capacity:

A. Abdominal distention
B. Asthma
C. Emphysema
D. Increasing age
E. Pulmonary fibrosis

Q99:

Regarding the anatomy of the bronchial tree:

A. The trachea bifurcates at the level of the T2 vertebral body
B. The right upper lobe bronchus has 3 divisions
C. The right middle lobe bronchus has 3 divisions
D. The right lower lobe bronchus has 5 divisions
E. The right main bronchus passes under the aortic arch

Q100:

Regarding how the central venous pressure waveform alters with different pathologies:

A. Atrio-ventricular junctional arrhythmias cause regular "canon a" waves
B. Pericardial tamponade increases the mean central venous pressure
C. Third degree atrioventricular block results in irregular "cannon a" waves
D. Tricuspid regurgitation results in loss of "c" wave and "x" descent
E. Tricuspid regurgitation results in prominent "v" waves

Q81:

A. T
B. T
C. F
D. T
E. F

- The vagus nerve arises from the nucleus ambiguous and nucleus tractus solitarius in the medulla. It exits the skull via the jugular foramen and travels down through the neck in the carotid sheath.
- The left vagus nerve runs behind the left brachiocephalic vein, then crosses the aortic root before descending behind the left lung root.
- The right vagus nerve descends in front of the right subclavian artery and then follows the trachea and passes behind the right lung root.
- Motor innervation to the diaphragm is supplied by the phrenic nerve which is derived from the C3 to 5 nerve roots.

Q82:

A. T
B. T
C. F
D. F
E. F

Regarding lung volumes:
- Functional residual capacity equals the residual volumes plus the expiratory reserve volume.
- Total lung volume equals the vital capacity plus residual volume.
- Closing capacity can be larger than the residual volume. When this occurs you get distal airway collapse, which can lead to altered ventilation and perfusion. Causes of an increased closing capacity

include: lying supine, increased intra-abdominal pressure and increasing age.

- Inspiratory reserve volume is usually larger than the expiratory reserve volume.
- Inspiratory capacity equals the inspiratory reserve volume plus the tidal volume.

Q83:
A. T
B. T
C. F
D. T
E. F

The stomach secretes approximately 1200-2500ml of gastric juice per day. The chief cells secrete pepsinogen, the parietal (oxyntic) cells secrete hydrogen ions and the G cells secrete gastrin. The stomach also contains mucus cells which secrete mucus to cover the gastric mucosa with a 0.6mm layer of mucus.

Parietal cells are stimulated to secrete acid by histamine, gastrin and acetylcholine.

Q84:
A. F
B. T
C. T
D. F
E. T

Thyroid hormone is secreted as tri-iodothyronine (T_3) and tetra-iodothyronine (T_4). The majority is secreted as T_4 and subsequently converted into T_3. Both T_3 and T_4 are active, but T_3 is much more active than T_4 (T_3 is considered to be 5 times more potent than T_4).

Once secreted, it can bind to numerous proteins in the plasma. It has the highest affinity for thyroid binding globulin but albumin has the highest thyroid hormone binding capacity. Less than 1% of thyroid hormone circulates in an unbound fashion.

Both T₃ and T₄ can be de-iodinated in the liver or kidney.

Q85:
A. T
B. T
C. F
D. F
E. T

Cardiovascular changes at term in pregnancy compared to the non-pregnant state include: an increase in cardiac output of 50%, an increase in heart rate of 25% and an increase in left ventricular end diastolic volume of 10%.

Pulmonary vascular resistance falls by 30% and systemic vascular resistance falls by 20%.

Q86:
A. T
B. T
C. F
D. F
E. T

Bile is produced in the liver at a rate of 1000ml per day. It contains bile salts and has a pH of 7-8. Bile salts are responsible for the emulsification of fat and the absorption of fat soluble vitamins (vitamins A, D, E and K). It is imperative that bile salts are reabsorbed from the small intestine (enterohepatic circulation), and the body is usually able to retain more than 90% of these salts.

Q87:
A. T
B. T
C. T
D. T
E. T

All the vitamin deficiencies listed are correctly paired to diseases that they are associated with. Vitamin B1 is also known as thiamine.

Q88:
A. T
B. F
C. T
D. T
E. F

Even though the brain only weighs approximately 1500g (2% of total body weight), it receives approximately 750mlmin^{-1} of blood, which is equivalent to 15% of cardiac output at rest.

Blood supply to the brain is derived from the internal carotid arteries and the vertebral arteries (which are derived from the subclavian arteries), which fuse to form the basilar artery. The basilar artery travels on the ventral aspect of the pons.

The circle of Willis theoretically enables a blood supply that can be maintained to all of the brain if a supplying artery is occluded.

The anterior cerebral artery supplies blood to the anterior 4/5 of the corpus callosum, not the middle cerebral artery.

Q89:
A. T
B. T
C. F
D. T
E. F

Type	Examples	Mechanism
I (Allergy, immediate)	Atopy Asthma Anaphylaxis	Fast response (occurs in minutes). IgE-mediated degranulation of mast cells following antigen binding and cross-linking of IgE.
II (Cytotoxic, antibody-dependent)	Rheumatic heart disease Thrombocytopenia Goodpasture's syndrome Autoimmune haemolytic anaemia	IgM/IgG antibody:antigen interaction on target cell surfaces.
III (Immune complex disease)	Arthus reaction Rheumatoid arthritis Serum sickness SLE	Immune-complex formation and deposition in tissues. Leads to local or systemic inflammatory reactions.
IV (Delayed-hypersensity)	Contact dermatitis Mantoux test Chronic transplant rejection	Sensitised T_H1 cells release cytokines that activate macrophages or cytotoxic T cells, which mediate direct cellular damage.
V (Autoimmune, receptor-mediated)	Grave's disease Myasthenia gravis	Antibodies produced to specific cell targets e.g. antibodies stimulate the thyroid-stimulating hormone receptor in Grave's disease.

Reference: Rajan, T.V. (2003). "The Gell-Coombs classification of hypersensitivity reactions: A re-interpretation". *Trends in Immunology.* 24 (7): 376-9.

Q90:
A. T
B. T
C. F
D. T
E. T

Prostaglandins are derived from arachidonic acid (which is derived from phospholipid or diacylglycerol). They all have 20 carbon atoms including a 5 carbon ring. Prostaglandins bind to receptors that induce varying G protein coupled responses.

$PGF_{2\alpha}$ is associated with uterine constriction and bronchoconstriction. A synthetic form (carboprost) is used in obstetric practice to induce uterine constriction in post partum haemorrhage.

Q91:
A. T
B. T
C. T
D. T
E. F

The major histocompatibility complex (MHC) forms an essential part of cell mediated immunity and is responsible for antigen presentation to T-helper and T-killer cells. The MHC class I molecule presents antigens to T-helper cells and MHC class II presents antigens to T-killer cells.

The expression of MHC molecules is co-dominant. All nucleated cells in the human body express MHC class I molecules but only professional antigen presenting cells such as dendritic cells, macrophages and B-cells express MHC class II molecules.

Q92:

A. F
B. F
C. T
D. T
E. T

The radial nerve is derived from the posterior cord of the brachial plexus from the nerve roots C5, C6, C7, C8 and T1. The radial nerve innervates all the muscles of the posterior compartment of the arm (which are mainly extensors) and the triceps brachii muscle. Injury to the radial nerve can present as wrist drop.

Q93:

A. T
B. F
C. F
D. F
E. F

Maternal transfer of gasses to the foetus works on the concept of simple diffusion down a concentration gradient. Therefore, for oxygen to reach the foetus the arterial partial oxygen must be greater in the mother than the foetus. Also, for carbon dioxide to leave the foetus the partial pressure of carbon dioxide must be greater in the foetus than mother.

It is important to remember that the umbilical vein has a higher partial pressure of oxygen than the umbilical arteries and that the umbilical vein has a lower partial pressure of carbon dioxide than the umbilical arteries.

Q94:

A. T
B. T
C. T
D. F
E. T

To prevent inappropriate thrombosis, the body has several natural inhibitor pathways. One of the most important is the activation of protein C under the influence of the thrombomodulin-thrombin complex. Activated protein C is able to activate protein S and together they can inhibit the most potent clotting cascade factors (factors Va and VIIa). This is why patients with mutations in factor V (such as factor V leiden) are pro-thrombotic, because protein C and S cannot inhibit the activated form of factor V.

In addition, the body can activate plasminogen in the presence of tissue plasminogen activator to form plasmin. Plasmin is able to then directly lyse the clots formed by stable fibrin molecules. The action of plasmin can be inhibited by aprotinin and tranexamic acid.

Q95:

A. T
B. T
C. T
D. T
E. T

Mechanisms of placental transport include: simple diffusion (e.g. oxygen and carbon dioxide), facilitated diffusion (e.g. glucose), secondary active transport (e.g. amino acids), active transport (e.g. iron) and pinocytosis (e.g. immunoglobulins).

Q96:

A. T
B. T
C. F
D. F
E. F

The anterior lobe of the pituitary gland contains thyroid stimulating hormone, growth hormone, adrenocorticotrophic hormone, follicle stimulating hormone, luteinising hormone and prolactin. The posterior lobe contains vasopressin and oxytocin. Thyrotropin releasing hormone is produced in the hypothalamus.

Q97:

A. T
B. T
C. F
D. F
E. T

Vomiting is a highly complicated process that is controlled by the chemoreceptor trigger zone (CTZ), which is located in the area postrema near the fourth ventricle of the brain. It receives input from vagal afferent nerve fibres and multiple receptors that are located in the CTZ region (these receptors include opioid, dopaminergic, serotonergic, muscarinic and histaminergic receptors).

The afferent vagus nerve fibres are stimulated by chemoreceptors and mechanoreceptors in the gut which respond to either stretch or to the potential ingestion of toxic compounds. The efferent limb of the vomiting reflex is controlled by the motor fibres of the vagus nerve.

Q98:
A. F
B. T
C. T
D. F
E. F

Functional residual capacity (FRC) is the volume of gas remaining in the lungs at the end of a normal tidal volume breath (comprising the expiratory reserve volume and residual volume of the lung). It is increased by conditions such as asthma and emphysema. It is decreased by increasing age, abdominal distention, lying flat, obesity and pulmonary fibrosis.

Q99:
A. F
B. T
C. F
D. T
E. F

The trachea starts at the level of C6 (cricoid cartilage) and ends at the level of T4, where it bifurcates into the left and right main bronchus.

The right upper lobe has 3 divisions, the right middle lobe has 2 divisions and the right lower lobe has 5 divisions.

The left upper lobe has 5 divisions and the left lower lobe has 4 or 5 divisions.

The left main bronchus passes under the aortic arch.

Q100:
A. T
B. T
C. T
D. T
E. T

All the pathologies mentioned are correctly paired with the changes that could be expected on the central venous pressure waveform.

23305179R00059

Printed in Poland
by Amazon Fulfillment
Poland Sp. z o.o., Wrocław